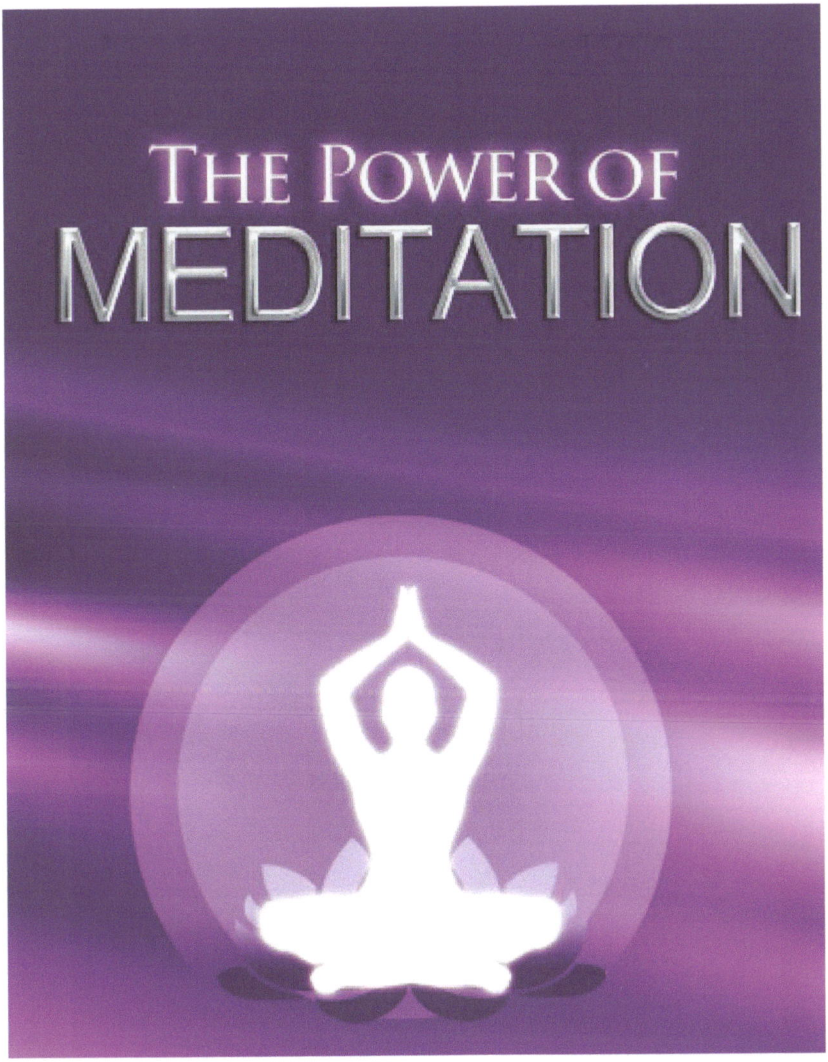

The Power of
MEDITATION

The Power of Meditation

Table of Contents

The Power of Meditation

<u>Chapter 1: Meditation and Success</u>

Mediation for the Modern Life

Somewhere in Silicon Valley, a group of computer programmers sit silently in a room together, legs crossed and eyes half-closed, listening to the sound of their own breath. Elsewhere, the owner of a small real estate company starts her day by breathing deeply and engaging in yoga poses. Still, elsewhere, a data entry specialist finishes his turkey sandwich and returns to his cubicle, puts on his headphones, and breathes deeply while listening to the sounds of bells and waterfalls.

Meditation looks different for different people, but one thing is for sure: it is quickly gaining popularity in Western culture. It has many professional and personal benefits including increased productivity, reduction of stress and depression, and reduction of troubling physical symptoms such as headaches and muscle tension, to name a few.

The word "meditation" often elicits images of devout men sitting silently in mystical temples far away. It can seem foreign and certainly something too far removed from daily life to have a practical application for business or even for personal gain. You may have preconceived notions about what meditation entails or cultural or spiritual beliefs which you feel may hinder you from participating in meditation. While meditation does have its roots in several spiritual practices, it is increasingly being recommended by Western medical professionals as research is bringing to light the multiple health benefits of regularly engaging in this form of focused relaxation.

The Power of Meditation

Regardless if you choose to meditate for spiritual reasons or for physical and mental health, meditation generally consists of the following elements:

- *A relaxing environment:* whether it is in the woods, by the lake, in a studio, or in your living room, mediation usually occurs in an environment that is physically comfortable and free from noisy distractions. Some people choose to sit on a cushion and focus on their breathing in complete silence while others may choose to lay on their beds and listen to relaxing music.

- *Posture or movement:* during mediation, the participant will generally sit in a specific posture, such as with the legs crossed, spine straight, and hands resting on the knees. Sometimes participants will lay down or engage in specific movements, such as with yoga or t'ai chi.

- *Focus:* while meditating, the participant will focus on a number of things from their simple breath, the feeling of energy moving through the body, an object, a value or ideal, or a word or phrase called a mantra.

- *An open mind:* during meditation, the participant allows their mind to let thoughts flow through their mind without judging them. Often times, the meditator will observe the thoughts instead of suppress them and then gently bring their focus back to the intended subject.

The Power of Meditation

How Meditation Increases Success

The idea of being successful, or being able to accomplish what you have set out to do or being able to achieve the state of mind you desire, is usually associated with words like "persistence," "patience," "hard work," and "goal-setting". Meditation most likely wouldn't even be one of the top hundred words associated with success. But it should be.

Think about it. If one activity, alone, could improve several aspects of your mind and your body at the same time, from problem-solving skills to general creativity to blood pressure, immunity, and headaches, wouldn't you think it could greatly contribute to your overall success in life? The healthier you are and the more empowered you feel, the more likely you will be to accomplish the goals you have set for yourself.

Making Meditation Work for You

While meditation can be a prolonged activity, it doesn't have to take hours of your day. Even a ten or fifteen minute session of meditation can provide some benefits of relaxation.

The following list serves as a reference for different kinds of meditative practices. Choose one or two that you think you might enjoy and incorporate them into your schedule. Many people prefer to meditate early in the morning before starting their day to help them start with a positive outlook. Others choose to meditate just before bed to help them relieve anxious thoughts and drift off to sleep peacefully. A few meditative exercises are detailed later in Chapter 3: The Practice of Meditation.

The Power of Meditation

- *Deep Breathing or Breath Focus:* Involves closing your eyes and focusing all of your attention on the experience of your breath filling your lungs and leaving your body. This is the basis of most meditative practices and many methods build upon this.

- *Body Scanning:* This method is used primarily for relaxation. It involves paying attention to different parts of your body in sequence, allowing yourself to tense and then relax each part, paying attention to how each part feels during the process.

- *Energy Focus:* Focusing your attention on the energy that flows through you and finding a sense of being "centered" or "grounded," meaning a place of relaxed and empowered wholeness. May also involve the use of "chakras" or centers of energy as dictated in the Hindu traditions.

- *Gazing:* This is a variation of the Breath Focus technique. Instead of having your eyes closed, you can choose to focus your gaze on an object.

- *Visualization:* Entails closing your eyes and focusing your attention on an image of a peaceful place, such as a beach, a mountain, or a favorite hiking trail.

- *Guided Imagery:* Involves listening to a teacher or a pre-recorded track to guide you through peaceful images and engage your senses.

The Power of Meditation

- *Mantra:* Involves repeating a word, syllable, or phrase many times, either in your mind or out loud.

- *Music:* Involves listening to soothing sounds of bells, harps, stringed instruments, wind instruments, and nature sounds while focusing on your breathing.

- *Yoga:* This exercise is actually a form of meditation, as each movement is carried out slowly and methodically, paying attention to the breath and energy in the body. It is especially effective when paired with a beautiful setting in nature or meditative music.

- *T'ai Chi:* A form of meditative martial arts that allows the user to focus attention on the inner energy flowing through the body.

- *Qi Gong:* Combines relaxation, meditation, movement, and breathing exercises to restore and maintain a sense of balance. Focuses on the Chinese concept of Qi, or energy, particularly concentrated around the spine, torso, and forehead.

- *Walking Meditation:* Walking can be used as a form of meditation when the user focuses attention on the feeling of movement, allowing all other thoughts to pass by. This is one of the most versatile practices because it can be completed while walking down the hall at work, on the sidewalk, or out in nature.

The Power of Meditation

- *Insight or Mindfulness Meditation:* Involves practicing mindfulness on the random stream of inner thoughts, feelings, and sensations as they flow by. It includes a focus on the present state of being as opposed to future or past events.

- *Positive Affirmations:* Entails focusing on the positive thoughts that will help you accomplish your goals. Examples include, "I am successful," "I am loved," "I am able to do this," or "I can do anything I set my mind to."

- *Reading Reflection or Quiet Time:* Involves reading a poem, sacred text, or scripture and reflecting upon its meaning or personal impact. Can also be paired with spoken word, sacred music, or journaling.

- *Movement Meditation:* Involves attaining a sense of groundedness or centeredness and then allowing your body to move in various ways, focusing on the feelings of your body.

Chapter 2: The Benefits of Meditation

The Benefits of Meditation for Business Owners and Entrepreneurs
If you have ever attempted to start your own business, you are probably
very familiar with the stress of working long hours, taking on increased
responsibilities, and trying to problem solve your way through unexpected
challenges. You might find yourself struggling to find time to eat three
square meals a day or sleep more than a few hours each night, let alone
adding something as indulgent as meditation.

Some stress is natural and unavoidable. Over time, however, increased
and prolonged exposure to stress will erode away the health of both body
and mind. It can lead to an array of symptoms including frequent
headaches, upset stomach and digestive issues, chest pain, difficulty
sleeping, and hypertension. Additionally, stress worsens the symptoms of
other diseases and can even slow recovery times from injury and illness.

Meditation, however, has so multiple benefits specifically for business
owners and entrepreneurs. After engaging in meditation, the mind and
body are relaxed, relieving the symptoms of stress. Meditation increases
the ability of the mind to engage in creative tasks, tasks which require
intense focus, and tasks which require problem solving. Additionally,
meditation helps your mind cope with barrage of information that can pass
through it in a given work day.

The Power of Meditation

It may seem difficult to justify taking time out of your busy schedule to "do nothing". But when you view meditation as a regular part of a healthy lifestyle and you consider the numerous mental and physical benefits; it's easy to understand why so many business owners choose to engage in it. Taking a little time to rest and recharge through meditation will increase the productivity and efficiency of your entire day.

Furthermore, after engaging in meditation, even the daily tasks of pouring a cup of tea, driving, or filing papers can become a form of meditative concentration as your mind is already geared up and ready to apply this newfound mindfulness to everyday situations.

Corporate Meditation and Employee Morale
Some businesses hire corporate meditation services to encourage their employees to engage in meditation together. Corporate meditation has a three-fold benefit for a company: it improves employee health and wellness, it increases employee productivity, and it increases employee morale.

Meditation results in reduced costs of employee absenteeism because employees can enjoy the health benefits of meditation including reduction of stress, injury, and illness. Employees will be less likely to call in sick because their bodies will be healthier. Additionally, employees who feel that their job is actually helping them to be more productive and healthier will report overall higher levels of job satisfaction, resulting in less employee turn over.

Meditation also increases productivity, especially for people whose professions require them to use their creative thinking skills or to concentrate for extended periods of time such as engineers, designers, architects, programmers, and artists. Additionally, meditation can help employees learn new tasks because it improves memory retention and general learning ability. When the mind is relaxed and free from distractions, it can work much more productively at the task at hand.

Meditation can help increase employee morale for several reasons. The first is that employees can develop a sense of emotional closeness by engaging in a shared experience together. Second, the process of relaxation can help lower emotional defenses which will in turn make the participants more likely to work well together on team projects and support each other under the pressures of deadlines, demands, and changes. Finally, employee morale can be increased by the introduction of a corporate meditation program as employees may feel that their employers care for their general well-being. Employees will find it easier to take pride in a company that takes pride in them.

Research studies are beginning to prove the benefits of corporate meditation programs. According to Project-Meditation.org, a Detroit-based chemical plant implemented a corporate meditation program. After just three years, they reported an 85% reduction in absenteeism, a 120% increase in overall productivity, a 70% reduction in injuries, and a whopping 520% increase in company profits.

The Benefits of Meditation for Personal Well-Being

The Power of Meditation

Meditation, especially when used as a regular part of a healthy lifestyle, has multiple benefits. When you review the list below, it will be easy to see why so many people are incorporating it into their professional and personal lives to help them achieve a greater sense of success. How many other activities can provide so many physical and mental benefits?

Physical Benefits

- Decreased heart rate, blood pressure, and cholesterol
- Improvements of symptoms of insomnia
- Reduction of symptoms of PMS
- Reduced thickness of artery walls, reducing risk of heart attack and stroke by 8 – 15%[1]
- Improvement of chronic pain symptoms
- Reduction of the distressing symptoms of asthma, allergies, depression, cancer, fatigue, and heart disease[2]
- Decreased muscle tension
- Improvements in levels of energy
- Increased immunity to fight off disease
- Reduction of free radicals, resulting in less tissue damage[3]
- Higher skin resiliency
- Slowing of the ageing process
- Decreased experiences of headaches and migraines
- Improvements in fertility as meditation helps regulate bodily hormones

---

[1] www.project-meditation.org
[2] www.mayoclinic.com/health/meditation/HQ01070
[3] www.ineedmotivation.com/blog/2008/05/100-benefits-of-meditation

The Power of Meditation

Mental Benefits

- Decreased anxiety and nervousness
- Increased feelings of independence and confidence
- Causes the brain to age more slowly by increasing grey matter in the brain[4]
- Increased creativity
- Increased ability to problem-solve
- Increased ability to concentrate
- Greater sense of self-awareness
- Reduction of negative thoughts
- Increased serotonin, resulting in improvements in mood and behavior
- Improved ability to learn new tasks
- Increased productivity
- Increased emotional stability
- Increased sense of intuition
- Increased ability to resist impulsive urges
- Increased job satisfaction
- Fewer distressing symptoms of mental illness
- Decreased feelings of aggression and road rage
- Improvements in listening skills
- Increased tolerance
- Increased ability to empathize with others and demonstrate compassion
- Increased sense of wisdom
- Ability to live in the present moment
- Increased ability to forgive others

---

[4] www.sciencedaily.com/releases/2005/11/051110215950

The Power of Meditation

- Increased sense of self-actualization or wholeness

Chapter 3: The Practice of Meditation

Preparing Body and Mind for Meditation

Meditation involves being intentional and mindful while placing your body in a comfortable position. Before you begin to engage in meditation, make sure that you have an allotted amount of time in which you will not be disturbed by phone calls or demands from family members or coworkers. Choose an area in which you feel safe and relaxed, with soft lighting and minimal noise. Make sure that your body is relieved by visiting the restroom, drinking water, and eating a snack or a meal beforehand so that bodily urges do not overwhelm you and distract you from your meditative exercises. You may even want to make sure that your body is clean and that your skin is moisturized so that you can feel most comfortable when gaining awareness of your body and so that discomforts do not overwhelm you.

Adjust the temperature of the room or wear appropriate clothing so that your body will be neither too hot nor too cold. Use a comfortable cushion with a soft fabric to sit upon.

If you are using music in your meditation, use something that you are familiar with which does not have any surprising clangs, screeches, or riffs. Put your music player on constant repeat so that you will not have to break your attention to start a new song.

The Meditative Posture

The Power of Meditation

While meditation does take several forms, from laying down to sitting to moving to balancing in various positions, many meditative exercises start with and can be completed with a simple sitting posture. This posture can be used for meditation involving mindfulness, breathing, imagery, gazing, prayer, and music among other things.

The meditative sitting posture is important because it allows the meditator to sit comfortably, allowing for good circulation and alertness while engaging in relaxation. Maintaining alertness is essential as meditation is not simply just relaxation, but it is also a mindful awareness.

Start by choosing a room or space that is free of distractions and that has a comfortable temperature. Turn off your cell phone and all other distractions. Wear clothes that are comfortable and that do not itch, shift, or dig into your sides.

Sit on a cushion on the floor. Or, if you choose, you can sit on a couch, an office chair, or a bed as long as it will allow you to comfortably maintain a strong posture.

Cross your legs in front of you, tilting your pelvis slightly forward to accentuate the natural curve of your spine. Distribute the pressure of your body evenly between your buttocks and your legs. If you are sitting in a chair, place both feet evenly on the floor.

Elongate your neck and your spine, allowing your head to rest in line with your shoulders. Slightly tuck your chin inward. Relax your jaw, your tongue, your eyes, and your brow. Let your shoulders rest in line with your hips. Allow your shoulders to fall back, opening your chest. Instead of crossing your legs, you could also bend your legs at the knees and gently press the soles of your feet together, tucking your heels in close to your pelvis. Also, you could engage in the "lotus" position, a traditional meditative posture, which involves crossing your legs and resting your right foot on your left thigh and your left foot on your right thigh.

Rest your arms on your lap or your knees, either with palms facing up or down, or with hands loosely cupped within each other. Alternately, you may choose to use a traditional form by connecting your index finger or your middle finger and thumb, forming a circle, and either turning your palms to face the sky with the back of your hands resting on your knees or turning your hands over, letting your palms rest on your knees. However you choose to place your hands, make sure they are supported and that your shoulders do not feel any strain from your posture.

Allow the breath to flow naturally in and out of the body, allowing the chest and belly to rise and fall as is comfortable. Allow your spine and shoulders to move with your breathing, ensuring that you are not sitting too rigidly. Take a few deep breaths into the upper chest, allowing your chest to open. Allow yourself to relax as you exhale, keeping a feeling of an opened chest as you do. You are now ready to engage in meditation.

Meditation Exercises
The following are a few simple modern meditative practices that you can easily incorporate into your daily schedule. These exercises are

appropriate for beginners and are easy enough that you can practice them in almost any environment, whether you are in the comfort of your living room, your office or cubicle at work, or sitting beside a river or fountain or in the pavilion of a beautiful garden.

Many of these exercises can be effective when used as little as ten or fifteen minutes per day. As you gain comfort with meditation, try engaging in it for longer, even as long as thirty minutes or an hour or more, when you are able to do so. Choose one or two that you think you might enjoy and give it a try.

- *Deep Breathing*: This is the core of most meditative practices. If you are unfamiliar with meditation, start here and do this meditation several times until you are comfortable with it before you move on to the different forms of meditation. Begin by finding a quiet, comfortable area. Turn off your cell phone and any other distractions. Place yourself in a meditative sitting posture. Focus all of your attention on your breathing.

  Notice how it sounds when you inhale and how it feels as your breath fills your lungs and then leaves your body through your nostrils. Breathe deeply and slowly. When your focus shifts to some mental distraction, slowly return your thoughts back to the simple act of breathing. Feel relief as your only task is to be quiet and listen to your breathing. Continue until you feel relaxed and rejuvenated.

The Power of Meditation

- *Music Meditation:* Choose a quiet place, free from distractions where you can comfortably listen to music. Turn on music which you find relaxing. Many people prefer to use instrumental music, especially ones that include the sounds of strings, bells, or nature. Engage in a meditative sitting posture and breathe deeply, relaxing your body and clearing your mind of worries and thoughts. Focus on the sounds and melodies of the music, allowing it to affect you. When your thoughts wander, return your attention to the music, breathing slowly and deeply.

- *Positive Affirmations:* Go to a place where you can feel safe and be uninterrupted from distractions. Engage in a meditative sitting posture and breathe deeply until you feel relaxed, clearing your mind of worries and fears. Think upon one or several positive affirmations about yourself. Here are some examples of positive affirmations you can use, or you can choose your own.

    - I am able to achieve anything upon which I set my mind.
    - I am doing work that I find enjoyable and fulfilling.
    - I am capable of achieving the success I desire.
    - I am competent and able to face any challenge this day.
    - I have the wisdom to make the best choices.
    - I feel the love of those who are not able to be physically near me.
    - I take pleasure in my own solitude.
    - I have the power to choose my own path.
    - I love and accept all of who I am.

- o I view my setbacks and losses as a gift.
- o I trust my intuition and my heart to guide me.
- o I am able to draw upon my inner strength and my inner light to guide me.
- o I am more than good enough.
- o I see the perfection in all my flaws.
- o The past has no power over me. The future will not control me.
- o All that I need will come to me.
- o I have a unique contribution and purpose in this world.
- o I am created in the image of God and am blessed with divine power and energy.
- o I am an heir to the abundance of God's kingdom.
- o The presence of God is around and within me.

- *Mantra Meditation:* Choose a mantra – a word, sound, phrase, or scripture upon which you would like to focus your attention. You might want to choose a quality that you want to incorporate into your life such as "love," "peace," or "forgiveness". Alternately, you might choose a favorite quote or scripture that has personal meaning. Once you have chosen your one word, sound, or phrase, go to a quiet, comfortable place, removing yourself from distractions and engaging in a meditative sitting posture. Start by breathing deeply. When you feel relaxed, say your word or phrase either to yourself mentally or out loud. Repeat your word several times, slowly. Meditate upon the meaning and impact of the word. Another variation of this technique can be involving the use of various prayer beads and prayers, using each bead to help you concentrate and focus on a prayer as you repeat it.

- *Body Scanning:* Go to a quiet, comfortable place and turn off your cell phone and other distractions. Place yourself in a laying posture for this exercise, resting upon your back with your arms and legs straight and your neck and spine elongated. You may choose to lay on a mat or on your bed. Engage in deep breathing, taking deep and slow breaths. First, notice what areas of your body are in contact with the mat or mattress. Focus on softening these areas by tuning into each part and relaxing it, whether you notice your hips or your head feeling pressure.

  Next, set a mental intention to leave all distracting thoughts or sounds and solely focus on your body. Agree to accept every feeling in your body, whether it is pain or relaxation. Focus your attention on various parts of your body, starting from your toes to the soles of your feet to your ankles all the way up to your head.

  Give each part of your body individual attention. Notice the various sensations of your body, whether you are feeling warmth, tension, pain, or relaxation. Imagine breathing relaxation, warmth, or acceptance into each part of your body. Finally, after you have paid attention to each part of your body, focus on how your body feels as a whole. Although traditional body scanning involves remaining still the entire session, you may also want to experiment with a variation by choosing to gently stretch or massage areas of your body that need to be relieved of tension as you engage in body scanning.

- *Visualization:* Go to a comfortable quiet place free from distractions. Engage in a meditative sitting posture. Start by breathing deeply, focusing on the sound and feeling of your breath and allowing your body to relax. When you feel relaxed, visualize an image of a peaceful place, either real or imaginary. Common places include beaches, mountains, or forests. Alternately, you could imagine a new place filled with fantastic creatures like unicorns and fairies or alien plant life. Focus on each sense. How does the place look? Imagine the visual details, focusing on each one. Imagine what you would feel, smell, taste, or hear in this location.

- *Guided Imagery:* Choose a pre-recorded guided imagery track or attend a guided imagery session with a therapist, teacher, or meditator as your guide. Many guided imagery sessions are available for free online through video services such as YouTube or through audio and video podcasts. Engage in a meditative sitting posture and breathe deeply. Listen to the instructions provided, visualizing each detail of the guided imagery as you listen.

- *Walking Meditation:* Choose a place to walk in which you will feel comfortable and safe, whether it is a sidewalk, a park, or a hiking trail. Instead of focusing on walking to exercise or reach a specific destination, focus simply on the feeling of movement and the soles of your feet pressing into the ground as they propel you forward. Slow down the pace of your walking so that you can focus on each movement of your legs, arms, and torso. Allow thoughts to pass through your mind without focusing on them, judging them, or holding onto them. Return your focus to the feeling of walking.

- *Reading Reflection or Quiet Time:* Find a quiet place, free of distractions. Silence your cell phone. Read a poem, a sacred text, or a scripture. If you like, read it several times and focus on each phrase independently. Then, read it again and focus on the meaning of the poem or phrase as a whole. Quietly reflect on the meaning of the passage and the impact upon your life. Listen to sacred music or spoken words. Write your thoughts in a journal, being sure not to judge any thoughts you may have. Alternately, you can choose to simply copy the text into your journal once or repetitively while breathing deeply as a means of concentrating, focusing upon, and memorizing the text.

- *Energy Focus:* Find a quiet place free of distractions and engage in a meditative sitting posture. Breathe deeply, focusing your attention on the sound and feeling of your breath entering and leaving your body. Focus your attention inward, gaining awareness of your feelings of being centered or grounded. The idea of being centered basically means returning your scattered thoughts and attention back to yourself and the space of your body. If you notice that your energy feels imbalanced or unfocused, try to refocus your attention to the energy at the core of your body. Alternately, you can also focus on different chakras, or areas of energy from Hindu tradition. The seven chakras are a complicated concept, but in short, they are:

- o The Crown Chakra – at the top of the head, this chakra is associated with spiritual connectedness, understanding, will, and the color violet or purple.
- o The Third Eye Chakra – slightly above the center of the eyes, this chakra is associated with intuition, psychic knowledge, and the color indigo.
- o The Throat Chakra – at the center of the throat near the collar bones, this chakra is associated with communication and the color blue.
- o The Heart Chakra – at the breast bone, this chakra is associated with matters of the heart, love, and emotions as well as the color green.
- o The Solar Plexus Chakra – at the diaphragm, between the breast bone and navel, this chakra is associated with intellect, cleansing, life force, wisdom, and the color yellow.
- o The Splenic Chakra – at the belly button, this chakra is associated with creativity and the color orange.
- o The Root Chakra – at the pelvic region, this chakra is associated with the earth, sexuality, and the color red.

- *Movement Meditation:* Go to a place where you can be free from distractions and turn off your cell phone. You may choose to do this exercise with relaxing music or in complete silence. Stand tall with your feet firmly planted on the ground, legs shoulder-width apart to form a strong base, and knees slightly bent. Align your head over your shoulders and your shoulders over your hips. Lengthen your spine and allow your shoulders to fall back, opening the chest.

Allow your arms to rest at your sides or bend them at the elbows, lightly pressing your palms together. Take several deep breaths, clearing your mind of all thoughts and focusing on your breathing. Continue to breathe deeply as you gain a sense of centeredness or groundedness. When you are ready, move your body slowly. There are several ways to engage in movement. You can simply stretch up to the sky or bend to the ground or allow your body to bend and sway in a snake like fashion or like a tree responding to the movements of the wind. You can start crouched on the floor, imagining that you are a flower blossoming, slowly and gently unfolding each and every petal until you are standing tall in the full light of the sunshine.

You can imagine that you are an animal, moving, stalking, and preening. If you are listening to music, you could pay attention the rhythms and swellings of the music, allowing yourself to dance in free-form as a response to the music. When you move, do not judge your movements, but accept the natural sway and rhythm of your body.

- *Gazing:* Choose an object which has particular meaning to you, whether it is a statue or picture of a deity or saint, an image, an object of nature such as a stone or a flower, or the light from a burning candle. Set the object up in front of you, slightly lower than eye level, in a quiet place free from distractions. Engage in a meditative sitting posture, close your eyes, and breathe deeply and slowly, focusing your mind.

Now, instead of leaving your eyes closed, open your eyes and focus your gaze upon the intended object. Try to keep your eyes open, without blinking for as long as possible. When you can no longer resist the urge to blink, close your eyes and picture the image of the object in your mind. Reflect upon the nature and meaning of the object, or simply allow it to capture your attention as you quiet your mind. Allow thoughts to flow through your mind without holding onto them or judging them. Return your focus to your object. If your focus wavers or the mental image of your object begins to fade, open your eyes, again, and repeat the gazing process until you need to blink, again.

A variation of this exercise uses colored candles, with each color representing different qualities[5]. Choose one color and focus on the qualities as you watch the candle burn. If you choose to use a candle flame, make sure you are in a place that is free from fans or breezes so that your flame does not extinguish or fluctuate wildly during your meditation.

- o White – clarity, wholeness, purity, innocence, and simplicity
- o Gold – wealth, prosperity, abundance, spirituality, higher ideals

---

[5] www.fragrantheart.com/cms/free-audio-meditations/spiritual-awareness/candle-gazing-meditation

The Power of Meditation

- o Silver – clairvoyance, personal transformation, the subconscious mind
- o Purple – commitment, reverence, connecting with the divine, spiritual development, and higher consciousness
- o Indigo – intuition, insight, wisdom, imagination, and clarity of thought
- o Blue – communication, self-expression, inspiration, creativity, relaxation, trust, and devotion
- o Turquoise – healing, independence, and protection
- o Green – Love, forgiveness, compassion, inspiration, hope, dedication, and freedom
- o Yellow – generosity, ethics, confidence, self-esteem, discipline, ambition, courage, inner power, and self-respect
- o Orange – sexual energy, sensuality, happiness, friendship, the ability to survive loss, and optimism
- o Red – survival, safety, connection to the physical world, courage, family relationships, physical strength, and vitality
- o Pink – loyalty, warmth, and empathy

www.ingramcontent.com/pod-product-compliance
Lightning Source LLC
Chambersburg PA
CBHW050925290526
45792CB00002B/889